Sleep – Rock Thy Brain

An appreciation of the wonders and mysteries of sleep

Daniel Crean
Publisher, Sleepdex

Daniel Crean

Daniel Crean

Daniel Crean

CONTENTS

Daniel Crean

1 LOVE SLEEP, NEED SLEEP

Fun, mysterious, beneficial, an important part of your life -- you should love sleep, too.

To use a modern metaphor – sleeping is like rebooting your brain and your body. We need to do it regularly to stay sane and healthy.

But sleep is more than that – more than housekeeping for the body. It's a pleasurable activity that can be indulged in for recreation.

Eudaimonia is an ancient Greek word that more or less meant "the good life.". It saw wisdom in balance and did not reduce human life to simple economic accounting the way we sometimes do now. Also translated as "human flourishing," eudaimonia should be incorporated into the design of our lives. Sleep is a vital part of that flourishing, both to enable us to accomplish more and as an end in itself.

The evolutionary reasons for sleep are a **mystery**. There are ideas, but no consensus theory on why nature makes us sleep. Sleep has more than one function, so there may be many reasons sleep arose. The biological benefits of sleep include:

- Repair of cell damage caused by daily life. Restoration of tissue and rejuvenation.

- Rest and energy conservation.

- Brain and memory reorganization. Reinforcing memory and learnings that formed during the day.

- Flushing of brain waste through the glymphatic system

The reorganization of the brain and rearrangement of synapses happens at a faster rate during sleep. That's apparently why we wake up feeling refreshed, more optimistic, and in a better mood. This is a bit of a puzzle. Exactly what is being refreshed and why we feel this way is not totally clear, but so much of human consciousness is not clear. The biochemical basis and neurology of nighttime sleep and daytime sleepiness remain to be fully discovered.

Sleep is an **active behavior**. We need to sleep long enough (quantity) and well enough (quality) to function well during waking hours. Nearly all physiological and behavioral functions in humans occur on a rhythmic basis, which in turn leads to dramatic diurnal (daytime-nighttime) rhythms in human performance capabilities. Without good sleep, our waking life suffers.

Insufficient sleep can lead to obesity, to chronic stress, to the premature onset of dementia and heart disease.

Poor sleep makes us less creative, less alert, and less able to handle the challenges of daily life. We are meaner people when we haven't had good sleep.

Medicine can help solve, or at least mitigate, the worst symptoms of sleep disorders. But it can take us only so far. To get more out of life, we should take charge of our own sleep habits.

The ancients saw sleep as a gift from the gods, and over the centuries there have been many myths and legends that have grown up around sleep. Modern science is making headway in figuring out the underlying neurology and biochemistry. But we should recognize the wisdom of the ancients, too. The classical Greeks, for instance, were less sure they were in control of the world than we are today.

"In Homer, people do not just go to sleep, as if that was something one could do; sleep itself is a sacred gift." – All Things Shining, Hubert Dreyfus and Sean Dorrance Kelly.

A more humble attitude toward life, perhaps, than we have today.

Mythological cosmologies had gods of sleep: Morpheus, Hypnos, etc. Tales of supernatural sleep – Sleeping Beauty, long-sleeping dragons and sprites – were told, and sleep was a transition station between our waking world and another strange, often magical world.

Sleepdex

This book grew out of the Sleepdex website, available on the web at www.sleepdex.org. The websites contains over 300 pages of researched information about sleep science and practices. It was written to be both accurate and accessible to readers who are not scientists or doctors.

The broader Sleepdex movement is about getting people to understand sleep and embrace it. We reject the dismissal of sleep as wasted time. We believe that ordinary individuals can enhance the qualities of their lives by appreciating and celebrating sleep. We want to recognize sleep as a pleasurable and inexpensive activity – an indulgence, at times. Sleep is fun.

2 SLEEP IS GOOD AND GOOD FOR YOU!

Sleep is good for you, even when you are already healthy.

The immune system is stronger when you get regular sleep. Short sleep on a regular basis makes you more susceptible to infectious diseases. The effectiveness of the flu vaccine is lower when you get insufficient sleep.

Insufficient sleep puts your body under stress and results in higher levels of stress hormones in the bloodstream.

People are in better moods after a good night's sleep – sleep deprivation makes you grumpy.

The effect on mood is not just due to our general tendency to feel better when we feel stronger. It has been shown that the changes in brain chemistry after sleeping are similar to changes after taking antidepressant drugs.

Your brain consolidates memories during sleep and you need a night's sleep to really learn something. Memories are transferred from short-term to long-term storage during sleep and both factual knowledge and physical skills are learned in conjunction with sleep.

Creativity is also enhanced by sleep. Not just for artists, either; the ordinary person can come up with better ideas after a good sleep. You can think harder and more clearly when rested.

Breaking Down Sleep

Physiologists have a procedure called EEG (electroencephalography) that involves measuring electrical potential between different parts of the scalp. The measure of the potential difference over time can be plotted. Some might call these graphs brain waves, but strictly speaking they are not waves, just records of voltage fluctuations through the night.

If you look at the EEG over the course of the night, you can see patterns that correspond to different stages of sleep. **Stage 1** is the very beginning of sleep, after the transition from waking. The person can be awakened easily. In this stage, the eyes move slowly and muscle activity slows. In **stage 2**, eye movement stops and EEG waves become slower. When a person enters **stage 3**, extremely slow brain waves called delta waves are interspersed with smaller, faster waves. In **stage 4**, the brain produces delta waves almost exclusively. Sleep professionals differ about whether there is a stage 4, and some lump stages 3 and 4 together. Stages 1 and 2 are **light sleep** and stages 3 and 4 are **deep sleep**.

The final stage is called Rapid Eye Movement or **REM**, or even stage R. On the EEG this stage looks more like waking. REM sleep is quite different from the other stages (which lumped together can be referred to as Non-REM or NREM sleep) in terms of what goes on in the brain and body.

Mysteries

Sleep isn't totally *terra incognita*, but so much is unknown.

Do you know why you go to sleep every night? Not a smart-ass answer like "because I'm sleepy" but the underlying biological reasons? If you could figure that out you might win the Nobel Prize for Medicine and Physiology. Even the top scientists don't really know why humans and animals need to sleep. There are ideas and conjectures and an increasing amount of neuroscience, but no accepted theory that people agree to. This question is of interest to physical anthropologists, evolutionary biologists, psychiatrists, psychologists, and even dentists. We know why humans want to eat; we know why humans want to have sex. We don't know why humans sleep. But it is a fundamental drive.

Scientists still have an inadequate understanding of the physiology of sleep and the pathology of sleep disorders. Some of the mechanics of what happens when we sleep are known and even they have been discovered only in recent decades. Further, although depression and neurodegenerative diseases are associated with abnormal sleep, nobody knows if there is a cause-and-effect in place, and if so, which way it runs. Science continues to chip away at the mystery of sleep. But it is still a mystery.

It's fun to stay up late – Euphoria and Sleep Deprivation

Staying up past your regular bedtime is exciting and can feel slightly transgressive. The connection between short term sleep restriction and euphoria is an intriguing one, although not understood. People with bipolar disorder (formerly called manic depression) have manic phases during which they sleep little. Natural short sleepers often have an innate exuberance and have been found to be more positive and upbeat than long sleepers.

Sleep deprivation gives a lot of people a buzz or makes them giddy. Especially in the first night of staying up, many people experience elation. Indeed, sleep deprivation can even be a short-term way to reduce the effects of depression in some patients. Imaging research has shown that one night of sleep deprivation leads to an increase in brain dopamine levels. The cost may be negative emotions the next day, and repeated bouts of sleep deprivation are not good for you.

The Difference Between Sleep and Fatigue

Fatigue, also called tiredness, can result from overwork as well as inactivity and unhealthy eating. Medical situations (diseases, chemotherapy treatment, etc.) can result in fatigue. Sleepiness, also called drowsiness, often accompanies fatigue, but they are not the same. The way to recover from fatigue is to rest. The way to recover from sleepiness is to sleep. You can rest without sleeping. Chemicals or drugs like stimulants can counteract both fatigue and sleepiness for a short time.

One problem if you don't distinguish between fatigue and sleepiness: responding to the wrong signals. People with a history of insomnia might find themselves fatigued and go to bed. They lie awake in frustration. But they aren't really sleepy, they are fatigued.

Why You Sleep When You Do

The two-process model helps us understand sleep timing. In this model, each of us has a homeostatic process and a circadian process.

Homeostasis is the tendency of our bodies to maintain constancy. The body has mechanisms to maintain constant temperature, blood pH, weight, etc. If you go too far out of a range, the body returns itself back to normal. The homeostatic drive for sleep is easy to understand. During the day we build up a need for sleep. When we have been awake for a certain period of time (roughly 16 or 17 hours), our brains need to sleep. When we have just slept, our brains no longer have the need to sleep.

Circadian, which means "of the day", is a word to describe the daily-ness of our bodies. As diurnal animals, we tend to sleep at night and wake during the day. Physiological functions (cortisol levels, body temperature, blood pressure) rise and fall with regularity over the 24 hours. Cues from the environment – mostly light levels – entrain our body's circadian cycle to the Earth's cycle and hence to the rest of the ecosystem. We are programmed to sleep at night. Sleeping at night is not just a social convention – it's how humans sleep.

The circadian cycle affects our sleep propensity so we wake up when it is bright sunshine and sleep when it is dark. Even if we are short on sleep, the circadian cycle encourages us to get up in the morning, and even if we are not tired at all, the circadian cycle encourages us to sleep at night.

The two-process model sees the propensity to sleep as an interaction of these systems. Ideally, when we are in sync with the world and getting good sleep on a regular basis, we build up a need for sleep during the day (homeostatic process) and at night both the homeostatic process and circadian process make us sleepy. In the morning, our homeostatic process lets us get up (we are "recharged") and the circadian process also moves us to awaken.

When two processes get out of alignment – as often happens with shift workers, travelers, and people who intentionally sleep odd hours – problems can arise.

This diagram shows how the strength of sleep propensity from each process varies over the day. – Process C is the circadian process and Process S is the homeostatic process.

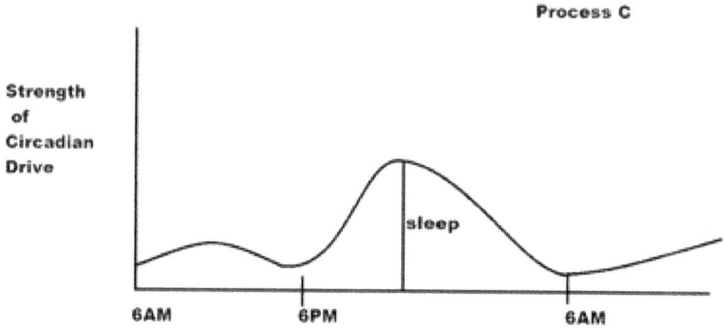

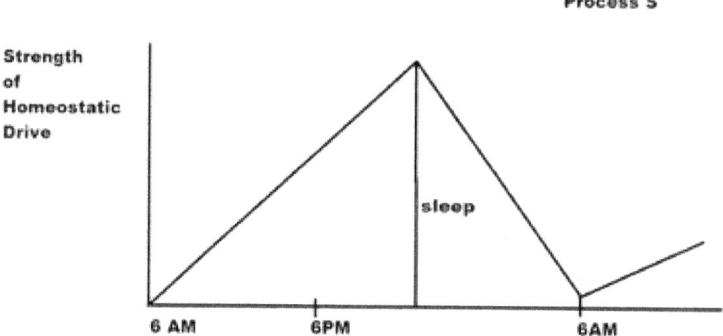

For more information

Learning and sleep – http://www.sleepdex.org/learning.htm

Creativity and sleep – http://www.sleepdex.org/creativity.htm

Two-process model – http://www.sleepdex.org/twoprocess.htm

3 LIGHT SLEEP, DEEP SLEEP, AND PARADOXICAL (REM) SLEEP

There are three types of sleep:

- light sleep

- deep sleep

- REM sleep

You experience all three in a night's slumber. You need all three. If there is any one type the middle-aged and older adult craves more of, it is deep sleep. Kids and young adults get lots of deep sleep. The rest of us can only envy them.

Light sleep

Light sleep encompasses stages 1 and 2 – mostly stage 2 because you spend little time in stage 1. It's called light sleep because you are easily awoken in this period and when you wake up from light sleep you don't feel too out of sorts. People woken from light sleep often claim they weren't sleeping.

The heart rate and respiratory rate are lower than in waking and the body regulates temperature as it does during waking. When people move around in bed they are probably in light sleep. The restlessness of some sleepers that results in tangled-up bedding occurs in light sleep. People who talk in their sleep do so during light sleep.

Light sleep is perceived subjectively as less refreshing than deep sleep or REM sleep, and this is part of what drives older people to complain about their sleep quality. Often called "shallow" sleep or "fast wave" sleep (because of how EEG readings look), light sleep gets a bad rap. The typical healthy adult spends 3 to 5 hours per night in light sleep.

Should we look down on light sleep? Is it a lightweight in the list of physiological phenomena? Wasted time? Just filler while your brain is moving between the more productive periods of deep sleep, REM, and waking?

No. Light sleep is useful and an important part of the circadian cycle and sleep architecture. The body rests during light sleep, and cell repair occurs, although perhaps not to the extent that collagen and muscle-building happen in deep sleep. Memory is "backed-up" in light sleep, to use a computer metaphor. Neuroscientists suspect that the brain transfers memories from short-term storage to long-term storage during Stage 2, making this form of sleep essential for learning. The "sleep spindles" that show up on EEG readings during light sleep are believed to indicate transmission of facts and memories from one section of the brain to another

People without serious sleep disorders usually have no problem getting enough light sleep. And when people are kept awake for an extended period, their subsequent recovery sleep contains substantial deep sleep and REM sleep, but light sleep is sacrificed -- which implies that this sort of sleep is less valuable to the brain. But we do know it has considerable value and nobody should dismiss light sleep.

Deep sleep

Deep sleep is the most refreshing sleep, as subjectively described by people after they wake up. Unfortunately, the older we get the less deep sleep we get.

Deep sleep is stage 3 sleep (or stages 3 and 4 under the classification system that includes a stage 4). This is also called **slow-wave sleep** to distinguish it from the fast-wave sleep of stage 2. (Slow-wave and fast-wave refer to EEG readings.) Deep, or heavy sleep, is so-called because it is more difficult to awaken people in this stage than in light sleep, and if woken suddenly from this stage, people have sleep inertia (i.e. grogginess.) People in deep sleep are less apt to wake in response to external stimuli like a loud sound than those in light sleep. Sleepers in deep sleep move their bodies less than in light sleep, although more than in REM sleep.

Deep sleep is a time of accelerated tissue repair. In children, this is a time of physical growth. Human growth hormone is released in the first deep sleep episode of the night, and the period is associated with rejuvenation. Common childhood sleep disorders such as nocturnal enuresis, night terrors, and sleepwalking happen during this period.

At some level, we crave deep sleep more than other types. If you stay up all night and go about your normal activities the next day, you have some sleep debt. But if allowed to sleep the following night as much as you need to feel refreshed, you will probably not double the time of your normal sleep. Rather, the sleep time is appended with an additional one-third to one-half of normal sleep period. So someone who regularly sleeps seven hours per night, may, after a missed night's sleep, go for ten hours before feeling refreshed. The interesting thing is the distribution of time among the stages during this recovery sleep. Pretty much all the lost deep sleep is recovered. The amount of deep sleep during this second night is about twice what it is in a normal night. Lengths of REM and light sleep are lower. It seems that the body chooses to conserve slow-wave sleep as much as possible, and it's more willing to sacrifice other stages of sleep.

REM (Paradoxical Sleep)

Only discovered in the 1950s, REM was originally thought to be the dream state. When people were awakened during REM they reported dreams. The rest of sleep time was classified as Non-REM (NREM), and for a long time experts suspected that REM was the really valuable phase of sleep, the part where our brains fixed themselves and NREM was mostly wasted unconscious time when the body was resting but the mind could just as soon be awake.

This turned out not to be true.

For one thing, dreams happen all throughout the night, not just during REM. Now the most "cinematic" dreams are indeed REM dreams. NREM dreams are often reported as flashes of images and emotion with no story or plot. If you have a dream that includes a narrative, it happened during REM. And the NREM phases are important for brain maintenance, too. They are not just downtime.

Weird thing about REM: you're paralyzed! Not totally, but the large skeletal muscles that move your arms and legs are paralyzed during this sleep stage. Scientists have even worked out how the nervous system shuts down these pathways. Good thing, too, or you might act out your dreams and that would be wild (and potentially dangerous to yourself and others in the house).

Your respiratory system works during REM, so it's not all muscles that are paralyzed. And if you look at a person who is in REM, you will see their eyelids fluttering. This is the origin of the term Rapid Eye Movement.

You might see a dog twitching its legs while asleep and hear someone say the dog is dreaming of chasing rabbits. Unlikely. Dogs and other mammals experience REM, too, and their large muscles are inactive during REM. A dog might dream of chasing a rabbit, but that dream probably happens when the dog's body is motionless. Twitching legs happen in NREM.

You might have heard that horses sleep while standing. True, but only to an extent. Horses can experience NREM sleep while standing. But they must lie down to enter REM sleep. The muscles required to stand would not remain flexed during REM.

Also called "paradoxical sleep," REM is almost a hybrid of waking and NREM sleep. Some neurons and brain areas are as active as during waking; others are silent or dormant. The EEG readings for REM look a lot like the readings for waking. Stages 1, 2, and 3 look considerably different from waking -- but, at first blush, REM and waking look alike. A trained technician can distinguish between the two states, but the similarity suggests waking and REM are on some level alike.

What is the purpose of REM sleep? Why did evolution give it to us? This is largely a mystery. Dreams may play a function for organization of the mind and allow us to rehearse scenarios or re-live situations. There is even a theory that REM is a sort of virtual reality program run by the brain. In this view, REM is a proto conscious state that helps us rehearse and mentally act out scenarios in a manner similar to how play helps us.

But dreams are not the only reason for REM. Even newborn babies who have little experience of the world spend a lot of time in REM. Indeed, even fetuses, who have never been outside their mothers' uteruses, experience REM. Are the fetuses dreaming in the sense that adults dream? They have no experience of the world, so the answer must be "no.". REM is about more than dreaming.

The course of sleep during the night

If you look at a hypnogram (a graph of the stages) you see the progression of stages through the night: 1, 2, 3, REM, back to 1. There is often a brief waking period at the end of REM. It might last less than a minute. Even if you think you slept the whole night through without waking, you probably did wake briefly, but went back to sleep so quickly the waking was forgotten. The people who don't experience these brief awakenings tend to be people recovering from sleep deprivation.

Hypnogram

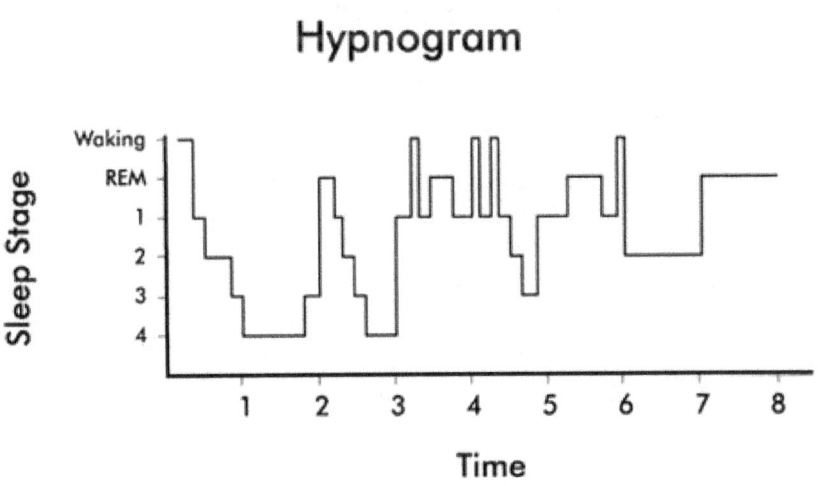

Another interesting thing is the length of time of each stage and how that changes through the night. Early in the night the deep sleep periods are longest and they shorten as the night progresses. Late in the sleep period (shortly before awakening,) REM periods increase in length. This suggests the body and brain are giving first priority to deep sleep and regard REM as more of a luxury that can be indulged in if there is sufficient time.

The cycle of progression through the stages and the length of time spent in each stage are collectively referred to as the sleep architecture. Drugs can alter the architecture and as a person ages the architecture changes.

Waking

Stage 0   (16 to 18 hours per day)

Eyes open, responsive to external stimuli, can hold intelligible conversation

NREM Sleep

Light Sleep (2 to 5 hours per night)

Stage 1 - Transition between waking and sleep. If awakened person will claim was never asleep

Stage 2 - Main body of light sleep. Memory consolidation. Synaptic pruning

Deep Sleep (1 to 3 hours per night)

Stages 3 and 4 - Slow waves on EEG readings. Release of growth hormone. Subjectively refreshing sleep.

REM Sleep

Stage R (90 to 120 min/night)

EEG readings similar to waking. Most vivid dreams happen in this stage. Body does not move.

Desirable Sleep

Newborn babies spend the day as follows:

8 hours awake

8 hours in deep sleep

8 hours in REM sleep

No time in light sleep! At the age of six weeks there is some detectable light sleep, and as the child grows the duration of light sleep increases while the duration of deep sleep, REM sleep, and total overall sleep time decrease. This continues to early adulthood.

By age thirty or so, the signs of middle age start to manifest in sleep patterns. This onset occurs at different ages in different people, but most 35-year-olds will admit they slept better when they were twenty-five, and it's not just because they have more stress in their lives. The degradation in sleep quality starts with a reduction in the length of deep sleep time. Remember, deep sleep is rejuvenating sleep. Paired with an increase in nighttime awakenings, the middle-aged person sees the good sleep of his or her youth disappearing.

Old age is marked by a further fragmentation in sleep and a reduction in REM sleep for many. It used to be thought that old people inevitably had poor sleep, but the new thinking is that healthy seniors can maintain good sleep. It's just that so many seniors have health issues and take medications that can cause insomnia, leading many to have trouble sleeping.

Do you want to "sleep like a baby?" Hell, yes, you want to. You probably don't want to sleep sixteen hours a day, but you do want to have more deep sleep, and perhaps more REM sleep.

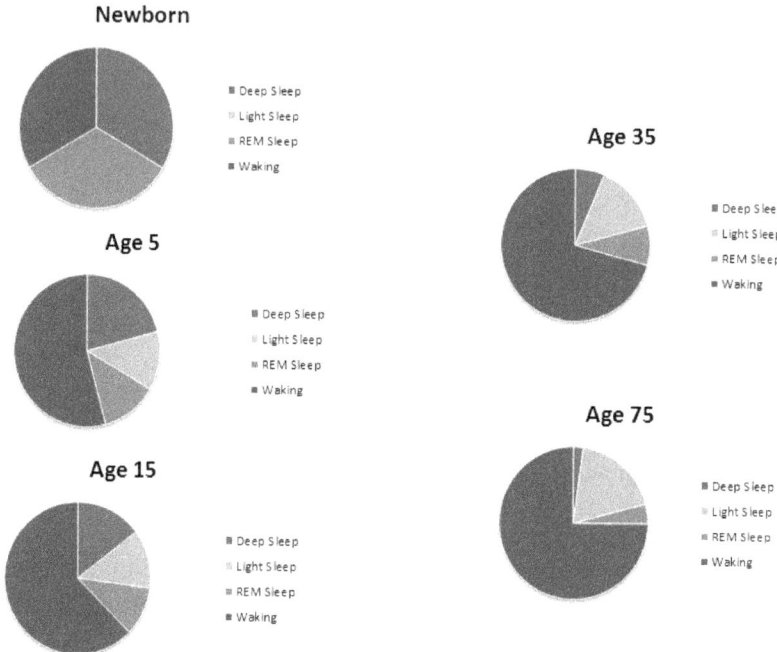

Beauty Sleep

Yes, it's a real thing! Sleep is a time of tissue repair and cell growth. Cell division happens throughout the day, but peaks around 2 am. The first deep sleep period of the night is when the pituitary releases a big pulse of human growth hormone. One reason staying up later than usual is bad for your health (and appearance) is that you miss that shot of human growth hormone. If you are used to getting to bed at 11 PM every time, your typical deep sleep period might start at 1 AM. If you stay up till 3 AM, you miss that first period and even though you get deep sleep when you eventually hit the sack, the hormone pulse doesn't come.

Further, changes in blood flow and body temperature regulation happen during the night, which can change the appearance of facial wrinkles. Combined with exercise (which itself promotes deep sleep) a regular sleep schedule can help adults remain young.

What does it mean to be "radiant?" It means the color of the skin moves closer to the color of blood. A radiator in a house or car movers hot liquid around to distribute heat, and so does the circulatory system move warm blood around and skin tone changes to affect body temperature. This is why some people appear more radiant just before bedtime or during sleep.

For more information

The Sleepdex website has more about:

Light sleep: http://www.sleepdex.org/light.htm

Deep sleep: http://www.sleepdex.org/deep.htm

REM sleep: http://www.sleepdex.org/rem.htm

Beauty sleep: http://www.sleepdex.org/beauty.htm

4 QUIRKS, PATTERNS, AND HACKING

Larkiness

Or to be more scientific: chronotypes. Humans are diurnal – active in the day and sleeping at night. But the time of sleep varies from person to person.

We all know "morning people" who are active and alert in the morning and "night people" who function better in the evenings. Without the demands of society, some people tend to be early risers and some late-to-bed and late-to-rise. Social cohesion and what your workplace, school, and family call for may take you out of your preferred time niche. There is a larkiness in us, though.

If taken to extremes, variation from social norms can be considered a sleep disorder. **Advanced phase sleep disorder** is when people get up and go to bed very early. **Delayed phase sleep disorder** is the opposite. Where to draw the lines of how far from the norms constitutes a sleep disorder is subjective, of course. And taking medicines (hypnotics, stimulants) to shift your natural larkiness to a socially acceptable sleep pattern is not a good idea in the long run. (It just results in poor sleep quality.) Some chronic insomniacs may just be extreme morning larks or night owls, and their insomnia is due to fitting into the standard sleep slot. These people feel like they have jet lag all the time.

Weird Hallucinations

Who needs mind-altering drugs when we have weird sleep? Hallucinations occur in the transition between waking and sleeping – more common when falling asleep than when waking up. (Contrary to what some people think, severe sleep deprivation does not produce hallucinations. When people are sleep deprived they might fall asleep and experience hallucinations during the transition to sleep, but as long as they stay awake, there are no hallucinations.)

Sleep paralysis (one phenomenon of the **hypnagogic state**), can feel strange and scary. It happens upon awakening from REM sleep. The muscles are paralyzed during REM and -- for one reason or another -- the paralysis persists for a moment or two upon awakening (this can happen during nighttime awakenings as well as in the morning). How bizarre is it when you are conscious but paralyzed, and when you have just come out of the dream state in REM? Imaginations can go wild and create stories about external forces working on the person in bed.

In centuries past this hypnagogic state may have been the source of nighttime visits by demons (succubi) and witches. There were many reports of people talking about witches sitting on their chest, which may be what their active minds extrapolated from feeling paralyzed in the dark and without markers back to reality. In recent decades reports of alien abductions follow the same pattern. People report the aliens are able to paralyze them in bed and perform experiments on them. A more plausible explanation is that these people are experiencing hypnagogia with hallucinations and their vivid imaginations are filling in the details with fictional stories. The "victim" does not necessarily think they are lying, and honestly thinks an external force (alien, demon) has had their way with them.

Bragging about how little sleep you get – the macho cult of deprivation

People love to brag about how hard they work or how much discomfort they put up with, and complaining (but really bragging) about a lack of sleep is a prime example. Subcultures with macho climates are susceptible to this. College students in schools known for their workload, medical interns, and special forces soldiers in the military fall to this self-aggrandizing boasting about lack of sleep.

One wag even called this phenomenon "sleep bulimia.". In the macho subcultures you often see (perhaps posted on doors) a triangle with the three corners labeled: sleep, study, social. With the admonition: "choose two.". In a world where being busy is a sign of status, we like to tell ourselves and others that we are too busy to sleep. We wear our ability to get by on a few hours of sleep a night like a badge of honor.

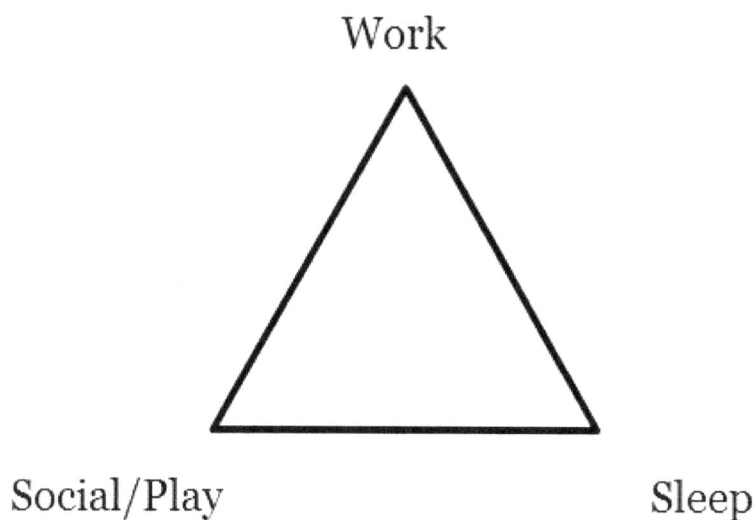

Work

Social/Play   Sleep

Choose Two

Often people try to cheat sleep during the workweek and make up for it on the weekends. Indeed, a large fraction of the working population does this to some extent and ends up with a weekend nap or late sleep-in on Saturday or Sunday. The diehards really try to push it and sleep only a few hours every night during the week. These diehards are almost all fooling themselves. Ergonomics, military, and human factors experts have found in study after study that performance declines quickly after only a little sleep deprivation. You might be able to get away with it for a day or two, but not for a whole week.

Sleep through the ages

Anthropologists who studied simpler cultures found sleep is often more fluid and responds to the environment and opportunity (e.g., is there food available?) more readily than in industrial societies with clocks.

You often hear people blame today's sleep patterns on modern technology. Before the industrial revolution, they say, people slept enough because they went to sleep when it was dark. Then came the electric light which allowed people to work and play into the night. After that came radio, television, the internet, and all manner of diversions to keep us up at night.

The evidence that electrification has been bad for sleep is less clear. Determining the schedules and patterns of daily life in the past is not easy. And it is wrong to assume that all pre-industrial societies had similar sleep patterns. Sleep practices and habits differ by season, latitude, population density, and primary economic activity. However, as best as historians can tell, it is true that people in Europe before 1850 slept more hours on an average night that they do today.

But that is not the same thing as saying modern humans are all sleep deprived. For one thing, the drive to sleep depends partly on context and environment. If it is dark and there is nothing to do, you will be more likely to go to sleep than if something interesting presents itself. People slept more before electricity because they had nothing better to do, while we do have things to do today. This is not a facetious explanation. Any serious examination of sleep must accept the observation that people sleep more when they are bored or feel less called upon to do work or pay attention to something.

Further, it is not clear that time spent in bed meant a time dedicated to sleep. Our modern ideal is that we go to sleep quickly after going to bed and leave the bed right after awakening. Indeed, the sleep hygiene practices advice experts offer (and which we endorse) calls for people to get out of bed if they cannot get to sleep. But not everyone follows that advice. And if you are not experiencing insomnia or a sleep disorder, you may wish to spend time in bed doing other things. This was even truer in the past when houses were smaller and the bed took up a greater percentage of the living space.

Bi-Phasic Sleep

So, records of sleep patterns may include this extra time in bed. Further, there is good evidence of widespread bi-phasic sleep practice in pre-industrial times. Bi-phasic sleep means the nightly sleep is split into two, roughly equal, periods. In between, the sleeper typically got out of bed and did housework, visited neighbors, read a book, etc. or stayed in bed and had sex. This middle period lasted an hour or even two hours. There are records of people speaking of First Sleep and Second Sleep.

Records from preindustrial Europe show a two-part split was more common in days before electricity. You probably know people even today who sleep like this: sleep regularly for half the night, get up and do things for an hour or two, and return to sleep for the second half of the night.

Are you one of those people who has persistent nighttime awakenings? You may wish to embrace a bi-phasic sleep pattern. If the first and second sleep periods go smoothly and are not fragmented it could be the best pattern for you. Plan to be up and out of bed for an hour or so during the night. Adjust your bedtime and morning rise time to ensure you get enough total sleep and find something to do during that mid-night wake period. If you embrace it and learn to live with it, you can sleep this way healthily and indefinitely. It's better than taking a sleeping pill to avoid that nighttime awakening every night.

Polyphasic Sleep

Polyphasic sleep is a strategy employed by some body hackers who want to spend more time awake. The aim is to have several shorter sleep periods throughout the 24-hour day, rather than one 8-hour sleep period through the night. Advocates claim that this allows the practitioner to sleep less total time, and therefore have more time for waking activities. The idea is that with more waking time, the person will be able to accomplish more productive work.

We are unaware of reports of women trying this sleep pattern. There are surely some, but the majority is decidedly male and decidedly young – say between the ages of twenty and thirty-five.

Why? It appears to appeal to some macho desire to overcome nature and not be beholden to either social conventions of time allocation or biology's call for a regular sleep pattern.

There are stories of geniuses such as Leonardo Da Vinci and Thomas Edison sleeping in a polyphasic pattern. Buckminster Fuller reportedly slept only thirty minutes every six hours, or a total of two hours per day. This has doubtlessly inspired others into thinking they can increase their productivity by employing polyphasic sleep. This type of sleep pattern is even called an Uberman's sleep schedule – *Übermensch* being the German word for Over-Man or Super-Man. Whether people are motivated to try polyphasic sleep because they suspect they are undiscovered geniuses or because they want to be more like those extraordinary individuals is unclear.

People stuck in extraordinary circumstances sometimes use polyphasic sleep if they cannot afford to be sleeping for long periods. Solitary open-ocean sailors in journeys lasting weeks use this technique. Astronauts in space missions and military personnel in certain endurance training regimens follow polyphasic sleep regimens.

Another name for this pattern is Dymaxion Sleep, which came from polymath Buckminster Fuller who applied the adjective *dymaxion* in many of his projects. (The term *dymaxion* comes from dynamic, maximum, and tension.) Others use the term Segmented Sleep.

Why are we down on polyphasic sleep? We're not so much down on it as skeptical. We celebrate sleep in all forms, and if you can get by on a polyphasic sleep routine and remain healthy and productive, more power to you. But not many people can do it successfully over an extended period.

Sleep as an Emergent Property

Borrowing from systems theory, we can see sleep as an emergent property of populations of local neural networks undergoing state transitions. *Emergence* is a word used to describe how complex systems arise from simpler interactions of small elements. Many properties in biology are emergent, and the concept finds its way to explanations of many phenomena including swarming behavior of insects and the movement of stock prices.

That's why we can speak of a person or animal being asleep or awake, even though there are so many neurons in the brain. When enough sections of the brain are in this sleep-like state, the person can be said to be asleep. Falling asleep is a state shift for the network.

That is also why tinkering with sleep is fraught with dangers and it is so hard to understand the physiology of sleep and to affect it through medicines without causing other problems.

5 TROUBLED SLEEP

Insomnia is extremely common. Pretty much everybody has experienced it. Maybe it lasts a night or two. Maybe longer. Some people have insomnia all the time – chronic insomnia. There are many causes of insomnia and not all causes are understood.

Insomnia is so common it is often just called sleep problems, sleeplessness, or trouble sleeping. There are dozens of different sleep disorders, but insomnia is by far the most prevalent.

Today physiologists see most cases of insomnia as incidences of **hyperarousal**. If you think of the brain as a battlefield between a drive to sleep and a drive to wake, insomnia happens because the drive to wake is stronger, not because the propensity to sleep is weak.

One distinction is between **sleep onset insomnia** and **sleep maintenance insomnia**. Sleep onset insomnia is when it takes a long time to get to sleep, when you are lying in bed just waiting and hoping for sleep. Sleep maintenance insomnia is when you get to sleep but then awaken, often several times during the night, and have trouble getting back to sleep.

Another distinction is between primary and secondary insomnia. **Primary insomnia** is when the insomnia is the main health complaint with no apparent other illness or cause.

Secondary insomnia is trouble sleeping caused by other illnesses or conditions in the body. Pain, colds and a stuffed up nose, substances (even caffeine as well as prescription and other drugs), mental illness (including mild depression), and a host of other situations can cause insomnia. If you eliminate or suppress the cause, you eliminate or alleviate the insomnia. At one time the medical profession regarded all forms of insomnia as secondary insomnia, and doctors were encouraged to always look for the underlying cause of the sleeplessness. To say that a patient had 'just' insomnia was to give up and not probe deeply enough for other conditions that were causing the insomnia. The mindset has changed, and now primary insomnia is recognized as a real thing doctors should take seriously.

A final means of categorizing insomnia is by the length of time the insomnia persists. Medical diagnoses generally distinguish illnesses which are acute (short term and will probably clear up on its own) and chronic (long term). For insomnia, a third category called transient insomnia is recognized.

Transient insomnia – very short term sleeplessness that will clear up on its own. Caused by jet lag (changing time zones), nervousness about a special or stressful event, unusual life situations (e.g. staying up late for a night or two, pulling an all-nighter in college or at work). When normal conditions return to the person's life, the insomnia disappears.

Acute insomnia – short term (under a month).

Chronic insomnia – persists for over a month.

Formal diagnosis criteria written up by medical authorities cover only chronic insomnia. This might seem dumb at first, but it makes sense. A formal definition has to have some standard of criteria and too short a period of discomfort is not classified as an illness or disorder. However, doctors, patients, and society at large recognize a two-week bout of insomnia as real insomnia, no matter what the manuals say.

Excessive Daytime Sleepiness

Another important criterion for a formal diagnosis of insomnia is "excessive daytime sleepiness." This phrase might sound screwy but the term is used in medical literature. Excessive daytime sleepiness is the cause of much misery, lost productivity, and motor vehicle and industrial accidents. If you wake up during the night but do not have impairment or feel sleepy during the day, you do not have insomnia by the formal definition.

You might think this is all too subjective and relies on the patient's complaints. That's right. There is no laboratory test for insomnia, no biomarker or stuff floating around in the blood that can identify an insomniac. Behavior and the patient's self-assessment and reporting are what a doctor use to tell if there is chronic insomnia. The Multiple Sleep Latency Test measures how long it takes the subject to fall asleep and short times are suggestive of excessive daytime sleepiness.

There is a sleep clinic test called a polysomnograph, which monitors a person's body through a night. It is great for diagnosing sleep disorders such as apnea, and can identify low sleep efficiency and high sleep latency that may be symptoms of the insomnia, but it can form only part of a diagnosis. And most diagnoses of chronic insomnia do not involve polysomnographs.

Chronic Insomnia is Worse Than You Think

Chronic insomnia can be truly miserable and degrade the quality of life for many. It can have long-term health effects, increasing the risk for obesity, diabetes, mental illness, and perhaps even Alzheimer's disease. It is one of the biggest, if most underappreciated, health problems our society faces.

Chronic insomnia poses a challenge for doctors. They are discouraged from prescribing hypnotic drugs for the long term. (Doctors have discretion to do so if they feel it is warranted, but professional guidelines and the FDA labeling generally oppose long-term drug use.)

The pathophysiology of insomnia may be a hyperactivated or hyperaroused nervous system. If this is true, it explains partly the chronic nature. The arousal does not easily diminish and does not go down at night. Sufferers describe it as feeling they can't downshift. Hypnotic drugs induce sleep, but the next day the person feels unrefreshed. People feel the only way to really come down is to take a vacation, and indeed, vacations often "cure" chronic insomnia, at least for a short time.

This type of dilemma for the patient and doctor – that the insomnia can apparently be stopped only by a vacation – is tough. It is one reason people retire earlier than they otherwise would and one reason we at Sleepdex want to spread the word about good sleep. We want people to find a way to sleep better to make their waking lives better and more productive.

An illness, a disease, or a disorder?

Is insomnia a disease or a disorder or an illness? It's certainly an illness because anything that is uncomfortable or bothersome counts as an illness. Some illnesses are also diseases. On the question of whether insomnia is a disease or a disorder, we come down on the side of disorder, at least for primary insomnia. Some diseases are caused by infectious agents or parasites; some are due to lack of adequate nutrition or genes. Primary insomnia is not due to these causes.

A disorder is a functional abnormality. Disorders are sometimes kicked off by a pathogen or external trauma, but there does not need to be an infectious agent to keep the disorder going.

Diseases can often be cured. Disorders can usually not be cured, although medicine often provides techniques for managing them. This meshes with our experience of insomnia, which can be treated but often returns. Nobody thinks the sleeping pills cure the insomnia. The insomnia just disappears, while the pills help the person get through the rough patch.

Treatment for insomnia

Cognitive behavioral therapy is a fancy name for teaching people to approach sleep in a healthy manner. Study after study has found this is the best way to address insomnia, giving the most lasting results with the fewest side effects. It is, however, expensive in the short run and does not provide instant results.

The course and scope of the therapy varies greatly. Therapists might be psychiatrists, psychologists, or nurses. Like other forms of therapy, the patient must do his or her part, and the success of this method depends at least partly on adherence to the regimen the therapist recommends. Some internet-based therapy programs are becoming available. The advantage of these is that they are cheaper than paying a therapist.

CBT doesn't work for everyone, but nothing works for everyone.

Related to CBT is sleep restriction therapy. **Sleep restriction therapy** advises the patient to sleep only while in bed and slowly reduces the available bedtime. The idea is that with less available time, the brain tries to fit sleep in the narrower window. Sleep efficiency (the ratio of time spent asleep to time spent in bed) increases and there are fewer and less severe nighttime awakenings. You can work with a therapist or you can do it yourself if you are disciplined enough. There are systems you can get over the internet or phone apps or you can just use a sleep diary.

Good Sleep Hygiene

Whenever someone experiences insomnia, the first place to look for improvement should always be practices and behaviors associated with bedtime and sleep, and to the environment. Taken together, this is called Sleep Hygiene. It includes the darkness of the bedroom, noise levels, and temperature. The type of clothing the person wears to bed, and the sheets and blankets can be factors. Good sleep hygiene even includes going to bed at the same time every night and refraining from reading or watching television in bed. (Mattresses are not much of a factor in sleep hygiene. Despite what the mattress industry might lead you to believe, there is no evidence that expensive mattresses promote quality sleep. We have never come across a scientific investigation showing that they do, and we read a lot of scientific journal articles about sleep.)

Drugs

Responsible doctors generally advise that if you can avoid using drugs, you should. Sleep hygiene and CBT are the best ways to overcome insomnia. However, if you must resort to medicine, most doctors agree that they can be used.

Back in the bad old days the pills people took to get to sleep were *barbiturates*. Barbiturates were widely used through most of the 20th Century, and it was common for households to have a bottle in their medicine cabinet. These are today considered a more primitive medicine. They alter sleep architecture (all hypnotic medicines alter sleep architecture, but the newer ones don't do it so badly.)

Barbiturates are true depressants, and result in lower heart rate and slower breathing. They can be dangerous. People committed suicide by swallowing a bottle full of barbiturates. Accidental overdoses, sometimes resulting in death, were common. Today's sleeping pills are safer. You shouldn't overdose on them or take more than prescribed, but if you do, the results are unlikely to be as catastrophic as an overdose of barbiturates was.

Trivia: in the 1966 novel *Valley of the Dolls*, the women protagonists took pills. What kind of pills? Barbiturates. In the Rolling Stones song "Mother's Little Helper," also from 1966, the pill that "gets her through the day" is apparently a barbiturate.

The next generation of medicines used for insomnia were *benzodiazepines*. These were first introduced in the early 60s and took off in popularity in the 70s. The 1972 Lou Reed song "A Walk on the WIld SIde" refers to Valium, and Valium was the brand name of a benzodiazepine drug that was widely used in the 1970s.

Benzodiazepines promoted sleep by mimicking the neurotransmitter GABA in the brain. They had less of an overall depressant effect on the body and were less dangerous to the respiratory and cardiovascular systems. They displaced barbiturates as the go-to sleeping pills. Like all drugs, they had side effects, sometimes intolerable. And they were unfortunately habit-forming, so did not present an ideal solution for those with chronic insomnia.

Benzodiazepines are still used occasionally for insomnia today, but have mostly been displaced for this use. There are over a dozen benzodiazepine drugs on the market and they are still used for anxiety, among other things. The popular drug Xanax is a benzodiazepine.

In the 1980s new hypnotics hit the market. (Medicines intended to help you sleep are called hypnotics.) These new drugs worked somewhat like the benzodiazepines but they were more targeted. They hit the same biochemical receptors in brain neurons, but the doses needed to induce sleep were lower so the risk of dependence was less. The medical world started referring to these as "non-benzodiazepine hypnotics" which is a pretty lousy name. (Lots of things are not benzodiazepines.) Some of these were **Zolpidem** (sold under the brand name Ambien), **Zaleplon** (sold under the brand name **Sonata**), and **Eszopiclone** (brand name **Lunesta**). Although developed by different drug companies, these new compounds got names with the letter Z in them -- which led to these drugs being called *Z-drugs*. The Z-drug moniker is better than the ambiguous phrase non-benzodiazepine.

Even today, the Z-drugs are the go-to prescription hypnotic. Ramelteon (sold under the brand name **Rozerem**) is not a Z-drug. It is interesting because it works through a different neural pathway. Ramelteon is a *melatonin agonist*, meaning it more-or-less mimics the natural hormone melatonin which plays an important role in the circadian cycle. Drug companies are investigating other ways to affect the circadian cycle, and ramelteon may someday be considered one of a class of medicines called *chronobiotics*.

Over-the-counter medicines

Walk into any drug store and you will find boxes of "sleep aids." They should not be used lightly as they are real drugs, but they are safe enough that the FDA allows them to be sold to adults without a prescription. There are many brands of OTC sleep medicines, but the active ingredient in all of them is a drug in the class called *antihistamines*. (Antihistamines have other uses too, and you may hear of them being used to address allergic reactions to bee stings.)

What drug should you take?

Ideally you should try to not take any hypnotic and should try to solve insomnia by other means. If you must take a medicine, however, consult your doctor. The choice of an appropriate medicine for each individual depends on that person's overall health, other illnesses and diseases, age, and other medicines used. Don't forget about other drugs you're taking, because drug interaction is a concern when people take more than one medicine.

You might think prescription drugs are stronger than over-the-counter pills. That is incorrect. The OTC drugs, which are antihistamines, target different neuronal systems than the prescription drugs. Some people experience the prescription Z-drugs as "stronger" than antihistamines, but others experience antihistamines as stronger. By stronger, people mean one or more of several things: (1) made them get to sleep faster, (2) reduced nighttime awakenings, (3) increase grogginess in the morning, (4) increase feeling of pressure to sleep.

Responsible adults can use OTC medicines as they feel is warranted. (That's why the FDA approved these drugs for OTC sale). If you REALLY feel you need to take medicine for your insomnia, you probably want to start with an OTC remedy and see if this works. Consult your doctor.

Remember that all hypnotics alter sleep architecture and may have other subtle, unknown side effects in the body, so use all such drugs with caution. They can also be addictive or habit-forming. The addition can be physical and psychological. So these drugs are best used for acute, short-term insomnia. Quit them after a couple weeks. If you do use them for chronic insomnia, you probably should take periodic drug holidays and space out your medicine use. Talk to your doctor about this.

Hypersomnia – Sleeping too much

The opposite of insomnia is **hypersomnia**. The hypersomniac regularly sleeps longer than normal. How much longer gets you into hypersomnia territory is not exact and relies on the judgment of the doctors, but more than ten or eleven hours every day seems to be a rough boundary of hypersomnia. Like insomnia, hypersomnia is not much fun. It is often caused by brain injuries (for instance, from accidents or strokes). Some people have idiopathic insomnia, meaning there is no apparent cause and they are otherwise healthy.

There is no real treatment for hypersomnia other than stimulants, and prolonged use of stimulants can present problems for the body.

The Sleepdex website has more on

Insomnia – http://www.sleepdex.org/insomnia.htm and http://www.sleepdex.org/otherins.htm

Hypersomnia – http://www.sleepdex.org/hypersomnia.htm

6 MONKEY WRENCHES IN THE MECHANISM: OTHER SLEEP DISORDERS

The medical establishment defines dozens of sleep disorders. Some are not serious and are almost comical. Others can be serious and threaten health.

The **dyssomnias** are disorders of sleep or wakefulness, in contrast to **parasomnias**, which are problems in the sleep/wake transition

Dyssomnias include insomnia, which is by far the most prevalent sleep disorder, as well as apnea, narcolepsy, and restless legs syndrome.

Parasomnias are often odd. We don't mean to make light of sleep disorders, but they are rarely dangerous. Parasomnias include sleep walking, sleep talking, and wetting the bed. Some of the weird phenomena associated with the sleep state are parasomnias hallucinations, periodic limb movements, and hypnogogia.

Apnea

Apnea is when the sleeper repeatedly pauses breathing during the night. The heavier you are the more likely you are to experience apnea, although thin people can develop it, too.

Untreated apnea leads to altered energy metabolism and increases the risk for obesity and diabetes. It also produces microarousals during the night and unrefreshing sleep. Cutting the air off produces stress on the cardiovascular system. It's bad all around, and another reason to avoid obesity.

You know how lead poisoning is bad for adults, but even worse for growing children with developing nervous systems? Apnea is the same. Childhood apnea, which is becoming more common with increasing obesity rates, poses risk to the developing brains of young people.

Restless Legs Syndrome

Is this a real disorder, or an example of disease mongering? The urge to move the legs that hits millions of people is a real thing, for sure, but some experts doubt whether it should be classified as an illness or disease or disorder. However, RLS is included in official lists of sleep disorders. There are treatments, but they are pretty strong – the same drugs used for Parkinson's Disease. Whether these strong drugs are worth taking – with their side effects – to mitigate the symptoms of RLS is debatable, and a lot of experts answer "no."

Narcolepsy

Narcolepsy causes frequent daytime sleepiness and falling asleep spontaneously even if the afflicted person gets a normal amount of sleep at night. These "sleep attacks" can last from several seconds to more than 30 minutes and can include cataplexy (loss of muscle control during emotional situations), hallucinations and temporary paralysis upon awakening.

In the popular imagination, narcolepsy is often confused with cataplexy and sudden loss of muscle down and falling asleep. Most narcoleptics do not have cataplexy, and both narcolepsy and cataplexy come in varying degrees of severity. People who collapse all of the sudden are pretty rare.

Sleep Deprivation and Sleep Debt

If you don't get enough sleep, you build up some debt and repay it the next night with extra sleep.

Many sleep researchers believe that modern society suffers widespread chronic sleep deficit.

Others aren't so sure.

There's a folk understanding of sleep debt, when people haven't had enough sleep. The unarticulated idea is that this is somewhat like a financial account, and that a built-up debt must be repaid. Indeed, people do sleep longer on weekends than on weekdays. But the popular understanding of sleep debt is not wholly accurate.

For starters, it is not a straight balance. Even after serious sleep deprivation, most people usually need only two or three good nights' sleep to get back to normal. If you run short one hour per night for five nights in a row (say Sunday through Thursday), you don't necessarily need five extra hours on the weekend.

Another exaggeration or misconception, according to some sleep experts, is the idea that we as a society get a lot less sleep than we used to. The evidence on this is sketchy, and even if it is true, it is not evidence of widespread sleep deprivation. Individual needs for sleep are context-specific and opportunity-driven to some extent. If you are not hungry, but somebody puts a steaming bowl of spaghetti in front of you, you might start to feel hungry. The aroma and opportunity make you hungry. Similarly if you are in the dark with nothing to do, you might start to feel sleepy, even when you are well rested. The modern world offers more interesting diversions than were available in ancient times, so the brain has more reason to stay awake. Sleeping fewer hours is not hard evidence of chronic sleep deprivation.

Do you really have sleep debt?

People who claim they are suffering sleep debt often show no more daytime sleepiness than anyone else. This has been shown using the sleep latency and psychomotor vigilance tests. People might think they have sleep debt, but there is no objective external sign. And formal diagnosis of insomnia requires that the subject experience excessive sleepiness during the day to truly have clinical insomnia. This disconnect (between a belief based on subjective experience and formal scientific criteria) may reflect ignorance about our own sleep patterns and what happens at night. Without nighttime monitoring people don't honestly know how they sleep. Sleep is a mystery to even the sleeper. But it argues against reports of sleep deficit being as prevalent as some believe.

Loco? No.

Sleep deprivation does not make people mentally ill in any meaningful sense. Insomnia is a very common symptom of many mental illnesses, so confusion occasionally arises about cause and effect. But the experts do not feel that sleep deprivation causes psychosis or schizophrenia or depression or similar problems. "Visual misperceptions" happen to sleepy people, but these are not the same as hallucinations or waking dreams.

Torture and Brainwashing

Law enforcement professionals might employ forced sleep deprivation to get prisoners to talk – the idea being that tired people have lower resistance to truth telling. It's hard to lie when you're sleepy. The United Nations calls sleep deprivation a form of torture.

Forced sleep deprivation was a part of attempts to "brainwash" prisoners. The North Koreans employed it on American POWs in the Korean War and the CIA incorporated it into experiments with mind control. Brainwashing is now mostly discredited and the stuff of spy novels. There is evidence that sleep deprivation can result in false memories, although it does not appear that handlers can manage the process and implant memories they want to.

Screwing up your own sleep

Stimulants can cause sleep onset insomnia, although some people actually find coffee or Adderall improves the quality of their sleep. Alcohol may be a depressant, but it messes up the sleep cycle and even when the drinker gets to sleep rapidly the sleep is less refreshing.

Staying up past your bedtime can be fun and short-term sleep deprivation does produce a sense of euphoria, but doing this habitually is bad for you – the "burning the candle at both ends" phenomenon.

Zombies: Just Misunderstood People with Severe Insomnia?

How are zombies portrayed in popular film and television? It could be argued that they look like people with very serious insomnia. They never sleep and they walk around in a daze. Writing in Scientific American, Bora Zivkovic fancifully suggested the zombies have a severe circadian disorder in which their bodies are always switched to the daytime mode.

For more information

The Sleepdex website has more about:

Parasomnias – http://www.sleepdex.org/parasomnias.htm

Dyssomnias – http://www.sleepdex.org/dyssomnias.htm

7 SLEEP AND SOCIETY

Sleep is important not just for us all as individuals; it's important to society, too. Humans are social animals and you can't function optimally as a social being without enough sleep. Families and roommates get along better if everyone gets enough good sleep, workplaces function more smoothly and more productively if everyone is well rested, and there are fewer industrial accidents and traffic accidents if machine operators and drivers are alert and not sleep deprived.

Shift work sleep disorder

The demands of some jobs make some people awake and at work when biology and nature want them to be asleep. The resulting sleepiness during the work shift and trouble sleeping during the day are called shift work sleep disorder. It's a circadian disorder, in a way, similar to jet lag except it doesn't go away as fast as jet lag.

The symptoms are a slow-burning multi-threat of insomnia, excessive daytime (or work-time) sleepiness, and unrefreshing sleep.:

Some people claim they adjust to the night shift and don't experience problems after a few days of adjustment. Others never fully adjust.

Surveys show that a majority of shift workers complain of problem sleepiness on the job or insomnia at home. The particulars of the work schedule matter a lot. Working evenings (such as a retailer or restaurant) doesn't normally cause many problems if the employee is off by midnight. Bar workers often work later than that. The worst is in people who truly have to work overnight and are at work when the sun comes up the next morning. The length of the shift matters, too, as long shifts add tiredness to the circadian disruption the body experiences.

Treatment can include stimulants and hypnotic drugs (sleeping pills), but they are not good for you in the long run.

Workplace Accidents

Public health experts estimate that over 200,000 workplace accidents and errors per year can be traced at least partly to sleepiness in the US alone. While most of these accidents do not involve injuries, sleep disorders are something that workplace safety professionals worry about because of the potential for loss of property and human life.

Such well-known accidents as the Chernobyl nuclear accident and the Exxon Valdez spill may be tied to sleepiness. Workplace accidents pose threats to a host of people and organizations: the workers where the accident happens, including contractors and supplier personnel who may be on site, the owners or shareholders of the business, the people living in the area near the accident (especially in the case of hazardous materials releases), the first responders from the community called to react to the accident, and the government in the location of the accident which may be called upon to do things it can't do.

Pilots and truck drivers are required by law to be off the job after a certain period. Hospital workers usually escape legal restrictions, but sleepy nurses, doctors, and technicians notoriously cause accidents in hospitals, often with life-changing effects.

Today industry in the United States is a lot safer than it was decades ago. Legal and regulatory agency rules, fear of liability lawsuits, and general awareness has made things safer and we have industrial hygienists scurrying around working on health and safety. But even today both employers and employees need to watch for sleepiness on the job.

Employers

OSHA regulations and similar rules may mandate period breaks for factory workers operating heavy machinery. These breaks give the workers physical rest and, it is hoped, help increase their vigilance when the machines start rolling again. But breaks and shift limits can do only so much. The worker must still get adequate sleep when he or she is at home. Coming to work sleepy is asking for trouble.

Work schedules usually include regular rest days, which may or may not be Saturday and Sunday.

Foreman need to recognize drowsiness and reassign sleepy workers. This might bring them into conflict with the union steward, but good management requires working out a solution.

White collar workers may not have high-powered machinery in front of them, but they can nevertheless have accidents that hurt or pose a risk to themselves and others. And screw-ups by sleepy office workers with oversight over operations involving dangerous machines and materials can be deadly, too.

Lost Productivity

Sleepiness on the job reduces productivity and is another example of the loss of human potential that happens when people don't get adequate and refreshing sleep.

Even when workers don't show outward signs of sleepiness, their inadequate rest effectively lowers their IQ, their attention to detail, and their emotional intelligence needed to get along with others.

Workers are understandably reluctant to acknowledge to others that they are sleepy. They may even be reluctant to acknowledge to themselves. Telling others or showing others you are tired and not at your best harms your reputation in the organization and may lead to getting fired, or at least not promoted or given a decent raise. So people hide it.

How much does inadequate and poor sleep cost the economy? Nobody knows. Plenty of studies have been done trying to quantify the costs in different countries, but there is no agreed-upon method on how to do the accounting, and whatever accounting you use, someone could easily shoot holes in it. The people who do these studies want to stress that the cost is very large, which is something we can all agree upon. Let's just say that in the United States the cost runs into the tens of billions. Added to raw dollar numbers is the more qualitative Quality of Life factors that decline with daytime sleepiness and nighttime insomnia.

Drowsy Driving

Sleepy drivers are dangerous. More dangerous than drunk drivers? Depends on how sleepy and how drunk, but the risks are comparable. Many drivers arrested for driving while intoxicated (aka driving under the influence) are guilty of drowsy driving, too. Think about it. The DWI/DUI arrests happen often at night after a few hours at the bar. The driver is both drunk and sleepy. The police officer charges the driver with drunk driving instead of drowsy driving, because the laws are more favorable for a conviction. It is easier to prove drunk driving through a breath or blood test than it is to prove drowsy driving. Further, every jurisdiction has laws against drunk driving while only a few explicitly call out drowsy driving in their road rules. (Police can stop drowsy drivers under general reckless driving laws, but there is rarely a law against drowsy driving per se.)

A drunk driver with a high level of alcohol in his or her body can be arrested even if the driving is textbook perfect; you don't have to be swerving all over the road to be convicted of drunk driving. But drowsy drivers cannot be stopped and arrested if they are following the road rules. Bad behavior is the only indicator. There is no physiological marker of sleepiness, and even behavioral signs show up only in the right context. Once a driver sees the flashing lights of a police car in the rear-view mirror, the sleepiness disappears and adrenaline makes the driver seem wide awake during the patrolman interview.

So this is a problem for law enforcement.

This is also a problem for public health officials, public safety policy makers, and other trying to curb drowsy driving: nobody knows for sure how much drowsy driving is going on. Or how many accidents are caused. The National Highway Transportation Safety Administration estimates there are over 70,000 drowsy driving accidents in the US every year but they admit it is only an estimate.

Reducing the Risk

If legal options are limited, the way to address drowsy driving is with awareness.

The transportation industry knows of the problem of drowsy driving and the risk it poses to them in terms of liability (lawsuits) and public relations.

Truck driver associations have programs to raise awareness of drowsy driving. (Whether individual truckers, many of whom are individual contractors, heed these warnings is another question.) Large transportation companies usually take measures to reduce the incidence of sleep driving.

For individual drivers going to work in the morning while sleepy or in the midst of a long trip on lonely highways, awareness and humility is important. Knowing your limits and understanding the need for sleep can save your life.

Modern cars are "too good" in this respect. They are quiet and smooth and so comfortable they lull the driver to complacency and sleep. Nicely paved roads make the drive smooth and uneventful. It is no wonder that people fall asleep. Rural roads with little traffic are a bigger risk than urban roads because they are boring.

The hubris and overconfidence of drivers is also a problem. Young adults are more prone to falling asleep at the wheel for two reasons (1) their propensity to sleep can be greater (one reason young adults are good sleepers) and (2) they don't appreciate the dangers of the road and their own limits as well as older drivers do.

But hubris and overconfidence can affect drivers of any age. So can just plain not paying attention to your own sleepiness. If you're most concerned with getting to work in the morning, you probably don't even think about your sleep cycle. The Monday after the switch to Daylight Savings TIme (when we lose an hour) is notorious for drowsy driving.

What if you know you are experiencing drowsy driving, perhaps in the middle of a long trip? The Sleepdex website lists some countermeasures you can take to mitigate the drowsiness, but the best thing to do is to get off the road and get some sleep. Or better yet, plan in advance to avoid getting into trouble.

Other people in the car also have a responsibility to raise the red flag if they see the driver falling asleep or not being vigilant enough. You might get yelled at, you might get into an argument with the driver, but you have a responsibility to yourself, to the other people in the car, and to people in other vehicles on the road to do something.

"What is the most dangerous sleep disorder?" is a bar debate topic for sleep scientists. While apnea contributes to cardiovascular risk and REM Behavior Disorder can cause serious accidents in the bedroom, it could be argued that simple insomnia and sleeplessness is more of a danger to society as a whole because of the sheer number of people who are afflicted and because they lead to traffic accidents and industrial accidents.

Crankiness

Here's another social problem caused by inadequate sleep: people are crankier and less sociable when they are tired and/or sleepy. The resulting fraying in friendship and family relationships is nothing to dismiss off-hand. It's another example of lost human potential due to sleep problems and our society's failure to embrace and appreciate sleep.

Different people respond to sleep debt differently and this even shows up on tests of reaction speed. Some deal with insufficient sleep better than others. But it is safe to say that we all lose a little bit of emotional intelligence when we are tired.

How much would the divorce rate decline if we all got better sleep? Would domestic violence calls decline if people were better rested and more level-headed? Would individuals be able to earn more money if they weren't sleep deprived?

Anybody who thinks and cares about sleep reaches the conclusion that **Quality of Life** is affected by how well we sleep. Bad sleep = less Eudaimonia. As a public health problem, the effect of insomnia and other sleep disorders on the disposition of millions of people should not be discounted.

For more information

The Sleepdex website has more about:

Costs of Insomnia – http://www.sleepdex.org/costs.htm

Shift Work Sleep Disorder – http://www.sleepdex.org/shiftwork.htm

Drowsy Driving – http://www.sleepdex.org/drowsy-driving.htm

8 WAKING – THE FLIP SIDE TO SLEEP

One of the benefits of good sleep is being at your best when you are awake. Waking could be considered Stage 0 in the stages of sleep.

All other things being equal, the person with a good night's sleep behind them is better equipped to handle the world than the person who tossed and turned all night. Good sleepers are smarter, more emotionally balanced, and able to react faster. They can work harder and play harder.

It works both ways, too. The quality of waking affects how fast you can get to sleep at night. Exposure to interesting stimulation during the day keeps one from getting sleepy, in contrast to bored people who can become sleepy even with no deprivation.

Vigilance

Vigilance is a term for relaxed alertness and it has become a buzzword for a desired trait among the human performance community. The military, for instance, wants to find ways to make soldiers vigilant so they can perform at a high level when needed, spontaneously. Rest and sleep are needed to be vigilant.

Sleep researchers and enthusiasts are interested in how sleep quality and duration affect vigilance. Excessive daytime sleepiness, the hallmark of so many sleep disorders, is obviously detrimental to vigilance. So are microsleeps – one or two second sleep periods that afflict the sleep deprived.

If sleep is a mystery which scientists don't fully understand, the functions and performance of the waking brain are not a whole lot clearer. Behavioral tests are useful in judging how vigilant a person is at a given time. Predicting vigilance and crafting regimens to promote vigilance are harder.

"Attention", "arousal", "alertness", and vigilance are terms used to describe human mental stances. These do not map directly to brain states scientist can identify through imaging techniques. They overlap, too, and there is no firm consensus about what those terms mean. How the brain focuses attention is still a mystery, although neuroscientists are making progress at understanding it at a microscopic level

Sleepiness and sleep debt are not the same thing. Both, however, result in lower performance scores in reaction tests. Sleepy people are not as vigilant, not as mentally quick.

Figuring out who is sleepy

It would be great if we could find reliable markers of sleepiness and of vulnerability to performance decline in cases of extended waking. The military, for instance, would love to know which of its members can perform in extreme situations, as would operators of airlines and trucking lines. Chemical biomarkers for sleepiness don't exist.

Performance tests (e.g. the psychomotor vigilance test) can help identify who is sleepy or at least who is at a diminished mental capacity, but they reflect the person's state at the time the test is given. They are not useful at all in determining who is going to see further declines in the next hour or two. Individuals vary in how well they can stand up to sleep debt and there is no way to tell in advance who will decline in performance when up too long.

Wakefulness and Quality of Life

If insomnia makes us cranky and miserable, its effect is more on daytime awakening that on nighttime tossing and turning.

When psychologists try to measure Qualify of Life, it turns out that the scores correlate more with daytime symptoms than they do with nighttime inability to stay asleep. That's why test and trials of insomnia therapies focus on daytime sleepiness, in addition to things like sleep efficiency and sleep latency.

Life is not as good when we are always sleepy. Which is another reason the Sleepdex movement is important.

Physical Performance

Rested athletes are faster, more accurate, and have a quicker reaction time. Mild sleep deprivation does not negatively affect aerobic capacity, but it does affect reaction time. Post-exercise recovery with extra sleep accelerates the building of muscle, strength, and endurance.

Trainers recognize the benefits of sufficient and even long sleep for athletes in heavy training.

When exercise physiologists asked heavy training swimmers and football players to sleep 10 hours per night (a lot by any measure), they found significant improvement in performance.

For more information

The Sleepdex website has more about:

Vigilance – http://www.sleepdex.org/vigilance.htm

Benefits of Sleep – http://www.sleepdex.org/benefits.htm

Microsleep – http://www.sleepdex.org/microsleep.htm

The Multiple Sleep Latency Test – http://www.sleepdex.org/mslt.htm

9 FUN SLEEP

Naps

Sleeping is fun, and one of the most fun ways to sleep is daytime napping.

There are many ways of napping – different lengths, locations, and times of day. Some people have a regular nap in the afternoon (common among toddlers and retired people). Others have a catnap during their lunch breaks. Opportunity and time budgets play a big part in napping behavior.

Retired people take a lot of naps because they have less structured days than younger people, but those of all ages can take naps. A Pew Research Center survey found that 34% of U.S. adults nap on any given day. Among those past age 80, the percentage was 52%. Men are more likely to nap than women and regular exercisers are more likely to nap than sedentary people

What used to be called a catnap is now called a **power nap**. The word "power" makes it acceptable for working adults who think of themselves as on the top of their game and helps sell napping to people who might otherwise think of it as an activity for small children and old people.

Appetitive nappers and replacement nappers

Appetitive nappers can nap at almost any time, and do so often to "tune out" of their surroundings. Replacement nappers are trying to catch up on sleep. Appetitive nappers can nap even when not sleepy. Replacement nappers are usually not in the mental state or habit that allows them to sleep at will.

Daytime napping can improve mental performance in adults – naps can help us remember things we just learned -- but are naps better than an equivalent period of time spent awake just relaxing or watching television? Yes, it turns out. The time spent in napping is better for remembering than the time spent awake. Reaction times also shorten when people have taken a nap. Formal measures of vigilance and mental performance are higher.

Napping can be taken as a sign of *excessive daytime sleepiness*, a symptom of many sleep disorders, but this is an example of how the way we look at sleep differs depending on whether we are looking for pathologies or looking at human behavior for recreation. Recreational and appetitive naps are fun, and not a sign of a disorder.

Does napping during the day make it harder to sleep at night? Yes. All other things being equal, daytime napping will reduce the amount of sleep at night, and this often poses problems for people struggling to get and stay asleep Those attempting sleep restriction therapy should refrain from naps, but most of us have no reason to avoid a well-timed nap.

Recreational Sleep

Is sleeping fun? Sure! The extra half hour in bed in the morning, the mid-afternoon nap. Sleep can be one of life's true simple pleasures, available to people without regard for class or status or wealth. Did you know the Sun King of France – Louis XIV – had 413 beds and sometimes held court from bed?

Victorians regarded sleep as an indulgence to be frowned upon. Sleeping beyond eight hours a night was a sign of idleness or the deadly sin "sloth." To some extent we see this attitude prevalent in our 24-hour culture.

People frequently eat and drink well beyond their physical needs – the same applies to sleep. How do we know when enough is enough? There is no scientific or medical answer to that question.

Humans are not alone: most animals will also spend more time asleep when they are overfed or confined to cages and stables, or are otherwise bored. Calling someone who likes to sleep "lazy bones" is a slur.

If someone who appreciates fine food without overeating can be called a gourmand or epicurean, why can't we have a similar positive association for those who like and appreciate sleep?

Is there a less expensive form of recreation than sleep? Something that is available to all? We can't think of any.

The Sleepdex website has more about:

Power naps – http://www.sleepdex.org/naps.htm

Appetitive naps – http://www.sleepdex.org/napping.htm

The Smart Sleeper – http://www.sleepdex.org/smartsleeper.htm

10 TOWARD BETTER SLEEP

Sleep Hygiene

"Sleep hygiene" originally referred to the cleanliness of the sleeping environment, especially with regard to bedbugs.

In contemporary usage, **sleep hygiene** refers all the practices and habits that help you get restful sleep. This includes comfort of bedding, room temperature and light level, noise level, regular bedtimes, and how recently you ate and exercised before going to bed. Improvements in sleep hygiene offer an "easy win" in the search for better sleep, and should be the first thing you go after when sleep troubles show up.

The principles of sleep hygiene function as tips to getting better sleep:

- Control darkness, temperature, and sound levels to your comfort. Experiment to find the best levels for you.

- Wear comfortable clothing and use sheets and blankets to help you relax.

- Go to bed at the same time every night and get up at the same time every morning. Set and maintain a sleep schedule. Try to stick to it even on weekends and when life gets crazy.

- Avoid alcohol, caffeine, and nicotine close to bedtime.

- Develop a relaxing routine before bed.

- Don't lie in bed awake. If you can't fall asleep within 30 minutes, go to another room and do something restful until you feel tired. Don't read in bed. If you want to read, get out of bed and sit in a chair.

- Don't go to bed feeling hungry, but don't eat a big, heavy meal right before bedtime.

You don't HAVE to do any of this, of course. Whatever works for you, works. Try different things and see what works.

Quantified Self and Home Diagnostic Technology

The Quantified Self movement uses newer information technology to find and record physiological data. The bathroom scale may have been the earliest link in the quantified-self chain, and subsequent development of home diagnostic equipment for measuring body temperature and blood pressure and sugar levels pushed things along. Nowadays QS enthusiasts record all manner of data about their bodies and daily activities. Steps taken in a day, calories burned and consumed, and mood are recorded.

Some home technology on the market promises to provide insight into sleep behavior. The now-defunct Zeno was a headband device that purported to record sleep cycles through the night. Wristband actigraphy devices so the same and some double as exercise recorders. There are even mobile phone apps that record the movement of the mattress as a means of measuring sleep time and cycles. (The phone is placed on the mattress with the sleeper.) It is not clear how accurate or useful these devices are, but it is reasonable to hope they will get better.

What can you do with this information? It could be used to design experiments and to figure out what kind of daytime behavior, bedroom temperature, mattress type, etc., make sleep go better.

The Sleep Diary

Sleep diaries have been around for years and they can be effective even when used in a low-tech manner. The diary is a record (at one time on paper, now on paper or electronically) of sleep behavior. The person keeping the diary records bedtime and rising time, and any number of other observations, which may include

- How long it took to get to sleep

- How many nighttime awakenings and how long they were

- Subjective evaluation of sleep quality

- Evidence of nighttime sweating and movement

- Exercise levels the day before

- Alcohol consumed the day before

Sleep diaries can point to patterns and help identify problems that can be rectified. Doctors often ask their patients with troubled sleep to keep diaries. Even if your doctor doesn't request one, and even if you are sleeping fine, a diary can be a good thing to help you sleep better.

Focus on questions you have and experiment. Will adjusting bedroom temperature or light levels affect your sleep? Try it out and keep track for a couple of weeks. You might learn something. Is it better to hit the gym before work or in the evening? How this timing affects your sleep may be something you want to factor in your answer to that question.

The other great thing about sleep diaries is that they don't cost anything. Maybe the cost of a notebook if you want to use one. Or just type the info into your computer. No special app is necessary. To get the most out of a sleep diary you have to keep at it every day for a period of time sufficient to answer your question.

Bring Back Sleep Manners

"How did you sleep?" used to be a polite inquiry, like "how are you today?" Its decline in daily discourse reflects a reduction in the social recognition of the importance of sleep to happiness and well-being.

Sleep manners are an old idea that we should bring back.

Also called *sleep etiquette*, sleep manners means respecting the need and desirability of sleep. Sleep etiquette is sometimes used as a synonym for sleep hygiene – the practices that promote good sleep. However, we are using sleep manners and etiquette to refer to interpersonal, social relations. Respect for others should extend to their private time, including sleep.

Yawning is considered rude. People were supposed to cover their mouths when yawning in public. While this rule is still followed by some, it is less prevalent than it once was. Not yawning and not looking obviously sleepy is part of presenting yourself to others. It is also rude to blatantly and unceremoniously tell someone they look tired or sleepy.

Calling on the telephone after a certain time at night is impolite. This time varies with culture, but a norm exists in after which you should not call. If you don't know a person well, assume they go to bed early until you hear otherwise. Similarly, there is a socially accepted earliest time of day you should telephone someone, unless there is an emergency.

If you are in the house with a person trying to sleep, you have a social obligation to stay quiet. This means turning down or off the television and music. It means not running around the house, but walking softly. It means not walking in on a sleeping person suddenly and turning on the light.

Bedrooms should have heavy curtains or shades that can keep the light out. If you have guests over, offer them a dark, quiet, comfortable place to sleep, with sufficient covers. Sleep care is as important to being a host as offering a well-stocked refrigerator.

Another important part of manners is not making fun of or questioning another's sleep habits. Just because someone needs more or less sleep than you do, or is more of a morning lark or night owl than you are, does not mean you should question them or imply they are lazy or unusual. Daytime naps are becoming more common even in cultures without a heritage of siestas, so respect them.

School Start Times

The research showing teens are naturally late sleepers (and not just lazy) has led to a movement to delay start times for high schools. There is much resistance to this idea due to competing demands. Parents want their kids out of the house around the same they leave for work. Teens want to have their afternoons available for part-time jobs. School districts have limited bus fleets and want to use them for elementary, middle, and high schools and delaying the start of one type of school often means making another level start earlier.

However, there is much to be said for delaying start times as a social policy, and especially for the high schools. A few districts have adopted this policy as have some private schools.

A World of Better Sleepers

Could better sleep lead to a reduction in the divorce rate?

Higher productivity at work and around the home?

A higher subjective Quality of Life for millions?

Lower traffic accident rates?

Fewer industrial accidents?

More creative expression by millions of people?

Faster learning by students in our schools?

A better, more harmonious community?

Always better

The definition of health that informs medicine is: the state of being free from illness or injury.

Medicine is about getting sick people well.

The World Health Organization has a better definition: "Health is a state of complete physical, mental and social well-being and not merely the absence of disease or infirmity."

And the WHO definition of mental health is even closer to what we at Sleepdex are getting at: "Mental health is defined as a state of well-being in which every individual realizes his or her own potential, can cope with the normal stresses of life, can work productively and fruitfully, and is able to make a contribution to her or his community."

Sleep is obviously an integral part of this bigger definition of health. Sleep is a fruit of good health and is an enabler of the elements of good health. Sleep can help people cope with daily stresses and work productively and contribute to the community.

There has been a new paradigm in psychology in recent decades: positive psychology. Positive psychology is the study of happiness. Traditional psychology as a discipline focuses on problems and how to solve them or live with them. Positive psychology focuses on how to live better.

The Sleepdex movement is about causing a similar shift in mindset regarding sleep.

Let's imagine there were a scale of quality sleep from 0 to 5 with 0 being minimal and 5 being mind-roasting awesome. Negative numbers on the scale reflect sleep disorders.

Sleep medicine takes you from negative 3 to zero. Who takes you from zero to 5? You do.

Medicine is not particularly equipped to make decent sleepers into awesome sleepers.

So the Sleepdex movement isn't just about making up for a lack; it's about expanding the boundaries of what's possible. Better, richer, more complete.

Our Proposal: The Master Sleeper

What would it mean to be a **master sleeper**? Other fields of human endeavor are ones which appreciate high skill and admire the best and the hardest workers. We speak of chess masters, of elite runners, or concert pianists. We acknowledge that while in-born talent is a factor in overall performance, so is practice and dedication. The chess master was born with an ability to see patterns, but he or she learned top chess skills through thousands of games. The runner trains constantly. Many professions mandate continuing education for seasoned practitioners.

Why shouldn't we be able to become better sleepers? The ancient and defeatist notion that sleep is just something that happens to you – Sandman sprinkles dust in our eyes or the god of sleep Hypnos or Morpheus supernaturally enters our brains and switches the sleep switch to "on" – can't we get beyond that? By taking action, proactively preventing insomnia, and practicing best sleep practices, we may be able to become better sleepers.

Sloth as a sin

The "seven deadly sins" formulated by the medieval monks included Sloth. The Bible in Proverbs 6:9 includes the line: "How long will you sleep, O sluggard? When will you arise out of your sleep?" But a more nuanced understanding of sloth sees it as "disinclination to labor or work." This isn't the same as the desire for healthy sleep. On the contrary, a person can't do work without rest periods and no one can operate at top performance without adequate sleep.

The Puritan work ethic can be adhered to and respect still paid to the sleep needs of healthy humans. It is wrong to see sleep as a shameful activity. We at Sleepdex want to celebrate sleep as a good in itself.

11 IMPROVING SLEEP

Sleep: so easy and yet so difficult.

Here's some advice you might hear if you have trouble sleeping:

"Don't try so hard." That can be the paradox of falling asleep. If you think about it too much you can't do it. The ancient Greeks did not have the attitude that they could control the world the way we do. Writing about the Iliad and the Odyssey, Hubert Dreyfus and Sean Dorrance Kelley: "Sleep is a canonical event in Homer because it is a paradigm of an activity at which one cannot succeed by trying harder." (*All Things Shining*, 2001, page 75).

Which may be maddening if you are having trouble. Sounds like some kind of Zen aphorism, doesn't it?

But there are things you can do to coax sleep back into your life, if you are an insomniac. And even if you are free of sleep disorders, you can take measures to enhance your sleep. You may not be able to *control* it, but you can *influence* it.

Roadmap

Here's a plan:

1. Assess Yourself – Figure out how you are sleeping. Use a sleep diary or a home technology device. Set a benchmark.

2. Construct experiments – Brainstorm different factors that might help.you sleep better. Potential factors:

- Duration, intensity, and timing of exercise

- Size and time of dinner and any post dinner snacks

- Temperature in your bedroom

- Clothing you wear to bed

- Biphasic sleep pattern (get out of bed an hour in the middle of every night)

- Timing of bedtime, timing of alarm clock

3. Martial your resources – Commit to spending time and effort recording your efforts and results. Buy any needed materials (although we generally discourage spending major money on expensive beds.)

4. Get help from others. Enlist family members to your cause. They can chide you if you fail to keep your set bedtime. Social media can make you accountable. There are on-line communities where you can talk about your progress and share stories and advice with others. By announcing your goals to others you may have additional motivation. It's no different from an exercise regimen.

5. Brag about your love of sleep. Preach the gospel of sleep.

We end with another shout out to the ancient Greeks: the concept of **Arete** – meaning excellence, virtue, the habits of betterness.

That gets at some of what we mean by trying to always improve your sleep and to appreciate sleep.

12 THE SLEEPDEX MANIFESTO

Every movement needs a manifesto. Here's ours:

Better, Richer, Wholer Sleep

We love sleep.

Recreational sleep, sleep for refreshment, sleep to help us think better and play better when we are awake. Sleep for fun.

We reject the medicalization of sleep. Why should sleep be discussed only when something is wrong? Why can't we celebrate sleep?

We need medicine when our bodies are going wrong. But what about when our bodies are going right? Even good sleepers can do better.

Sleepiness is not a sign of weakness. It is not a moral failing.

The ancients saw sleep as a mystery and enmeshed it in myth. Sleep was a gift from the divine, or a curse. It could come upon a person like a thunderbolt sometimes, and was impossible to resist.

Modern science explains sleep – to an extent – but as a phenomenon we can still love it.

Why should the only people who care about sleep be the ones who complain about it? Why can't people WITHOUT sleep disorders celebrate and treasure their sleep?

Sleep can be a revolutionary act. A subversive act. Is it subversive to fall asleep and skip a trip to the mall? To not read that book or clean the house because you are sleeping?

Sleep should be inexpensive. Sleep can be an indulgence because it consumes time, not money. There is no reason to spend money on fancy mattresses or luxurious sheets.

Sleep should be respected. We should not equate the desire to sleep with laziness.

Naps are good. They are not an attempt to avoid good hard work. They let us work harder and better.

Sleep is part of *la dolce vita* – the good life. The ancient Greek thinkers had the concept of **Eudaimonia** – today sometimes equated with human flourishing. We think refreshing sleep can be a big part of Eudaimonia..

Sleep behavior and patterns can be individual. Physiologists can describe common sleep quantities and behaviors, but we recognize there is no right way to sleep for everyone. Whatever works for you is valid. The quality of sleep is subjective.

We endorse the Quantified Self movement for those who are into that sort of thing. Knowing your body and brain can help you live better.

APPENDIX - WHERE TO GO FOR MORE INFORMATION

This book came out of the Sleepdex website. Sleepdex (www.sleepdex.org) is the largest and most comprehensive English-language website devoted to sleep. Scientifically accurate, it is written to be accessible to the intelligent layman.

There are many fine websites and books about sleep. The US federal government, and governments and institutions around the world, continue to fund research.

Sleepdex sections and pages of interest

Demographic groups

Seniors and Sleep – http://www.sleepdex.org/seniors.htm

Women – http://www.sleepdex.org/women.htm

Adolescents – http://www.sleepdex.org/adolescent.htm

Young Children – http://www.sleepdex.org/children-insomnia.htm

Economics and Sleep – http://www.sleepdex.org/economics.htm

Sleep Disorders – http://www.sleepdex.org/sleep-disorders.htm

Insomnia – http://www.sleepdex.org/insomnia.htm

Pathology of Insomnia – http://www.sleepdex.org/patho.htm

Apnea – http://www.sleepdex.org/apnea.htm

Narcolepsy – http://www.sleepdex.org/narcolepsy.htm

Parsomnias Section – http://www.sleepdex.org/parasomnias.htm

Dyssomnias Section – http://www.sleepdex.org/dyssomnias.htm

Circadian Rhythm Disorder Section – http://www.sleepdex.org/circadianrsd.htm

Sleep Debt – http://www.sleepdex.org/debt.htm

Drowsy Driving Section – http://www.sleepdex.org/drowsy-driving.htm

Alcohol and Sleep – http://www.sleepdex.org/alcohol1.htm

Body weight and sleep – http://www.sleepdex.org/weight.htm

Other Good Websites

Eric E. Chudler's sleep page – explanation of neuroscience of sleep from a professor at Washington University (http://faculty.washington.edu/chudler/sleep.html)

Harvard Medical School's Healthy Sleep – (http://healthysleep.med.harvard.edu/)

University of Maryland Sleep Disorders Center – (http://umm.edu/programs/sleep/health/sleep-disorders/adult)

National Center on Sleep Disorders Research – federal government's website contains substantial information on sleep – (http://www.nhlbi.nih.gov/about/org/ncsdr/)

Brain Basics: Understanding Sleep – National Institute of Neurological Disorders and Strokes – http://www.ninds.nih.gov/disorders/brain_basics/understanding_sleep.htm

Sleeping Well – from the Royal College of Psychiatrists – (http://www.rcpsych.ac.uk/mentalhealthinfoforall/problems/sleepproblems/sleepingwell.aspx)

Books about Sleep

We read these books and can recommend them. We have no financial connection to any of them and do not get any money from recommending them.

Say Good Night to Insomnia – Gregg D. Jacobs – 1998

Jacobs discourages use of drugs and stresses cognitive behavior therapy, reducing stress, and developing good habits conducive to sleep.

Coping with Sleep Disorders – Carolyn Simpson – 1996

Short and easy to read.

Sleepfaring – Jim Horne – 2006

We're big fans of Jim Horne who works as director of the Sleep Research Centre at Loughborough University. This book is both practical and philosophical and contains tremendously interesting ideas.

Sleep to Save Your Life – Gerard T. Lombardo – 2005 – Despite the hyperbolic title, pretty down-to-earth.

The Harvard Medical School Guide to A Good Night's Sleep – Lawrence J. Epstein – 2007

The Promise of Sleep – William C. Dement – 1999

- Long and expansive in coverage from one of the foremost sleep researchers of the past 40 years.

Sleep – A Groundbreaking Guide to the Mysteries, the Problems, and the Solutions – Carlos Schenck – 2007

Sleep – A Very Short Introduction – Steven W. Lockley and Russell G. Foster – 2012 – Very good

ABOUT THE AUTHOR

Daniel Crean is editor-in-chief and publisher of the Sleepdex website.